ASHLEY PERKINS

Lazy Keto. The Simple Guide to lose weight the Lazy way.

How I lost over 70 pounds with these few easy steps.

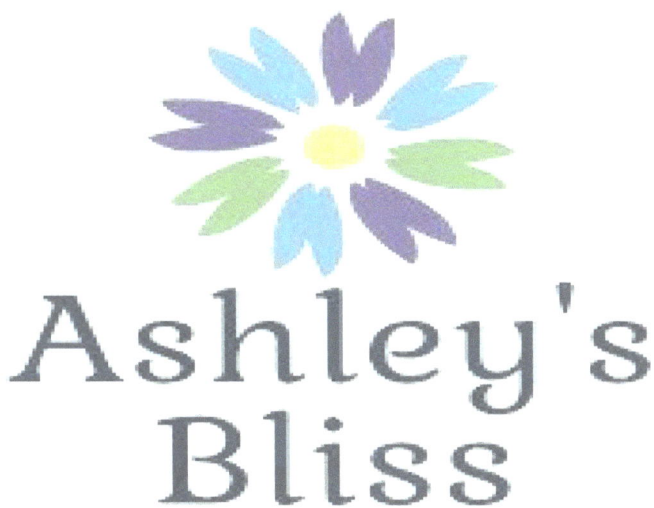

Ashley's Bliss

Copyright

First edition

This book was professionally typeset on Reedsy.
Find out more at reedsy.com

I dedicate this to my beautiful, loving family, who I love very dearly. To my friends who support me no matter what. To my love ones who motivate me every day to be a better person Ray and Paris.

Contents

Background — 1

So, What is this Keto Diet? — 3

How To Get Into Ketosis, The Lazy Way — 6

Simple Signs That You Are In Ketosis Yay!! — 9

What is the Keto Flu? — 11

The Cure for the Keto Flu — 13

Please don't tell me, I have to work out to lose weight? — 15

The Overall Goal — 18

Food List — 21

Weight Loss Journey Photos Before — 23

Weight Loss Journey Photos After & Current — 32

Epilogue — 43

About the Author — 44

Background

At that point I was hopeless, miserable, and thought
I will probably look like this forever.

Before starting my Lazy Keto Journey, I was all out of options. I tried all different types of diets that just did not work. If you can name it, I probably tried it, to no success. I was considered clinically obese, weighing over 230 pounds a size 16 pushing 18 with a BMI of over 36. I was at the highest weight in my life due to my poor eating habits and never having the time or energy to go to the gym. I swore to myself that I was going to start fresh the next day and go to that gym, but never did. At that point I was hopeless, miserable, and thought I will probably look like this forever and maybe, It was probably best to throw out those clothes I been hoarding in my closet from my early twenties because there was no chance, I was going to get back into those skinny jeans again!

One day, someone told me about this Keto diet, and I thought, hey Why not? Everything else I tried did not work, so why not give this one a go right? Who would have known, that this Keto thing would change my life for the better. So you might be thinking, "So you are saying, that I can do this Keto thing without much effort and lose weight?" Yes, it's very true! If I can lose over 70 pounds on this simple yet lazy way then, you can too.

Today, I can not only fit into my old skinny clothes, and those skinny jeans, that I almost threw away but I now can wear even smaller sizes (Mind Blown!) By following these simple steps, I will guide you through my lazy Keto way that will change and benefit your life forever, so let's get started on our lazy but awesome Keto Journey!

So, what is this this Keto Diet?

Yes, the rumors are true, you really can eat bacon
on Keto sweeeet!

The **Ketogenic** diet is a low carb diet, similar to the Atkins diet but you can actually eat some fruits and most dairy products on Keto Yay!!! With the Ketogenic diet or Keto for short, you actually get calories from protein and fats (yes, the rumor is true, you really can have bacon on this diet sweeet!!) and low carbohydrates. When you lower your carbohydrates to under 50 net carbs a day, your body in turn, burns unwanted stored up fat by making your body dependent on fat for energy not carbs.

Ketosis is when your fat stores are broken down to produce energy, also called ketones a type of acid. When you're in Ketosis, your body is forced to burn your fat (I know its amazing right?). The goals on Keto is to get into Ketosis and to stay in it, by adapting to a low carb lifestyle. In order to start seeing results right away, you want to be in Ketosis. It usually takes about two to seven days for your body to get into Ketosis the natural way. However, there are some supplements out there that can help you get into Ketosis a lot sooner, which I will go in further detail (It's a little secret ssshhh!).

There are numerous benefits to being in Ketosis and having a Keto Life style. The number one benefit is the weight loss (obviously). In the first week of starting Keto, most people tend to see some weight loss success. During my very first week, I lost ten pounds. Granted some of that was probably water weight but hey ten pounds is ten pounds am I right? When I saw that this Keto thing actually worked for me, it was the motivational boost that I desperately needed, to keep me going on my weight loss Journey. I hope when you see your first week's results, it can also be that motivator for you (that and I will be cheering for you every step of your awesome journey!).

Some of the other amazing benefits for being on Keto and having a Keto life style is that you will have more energy. Before starting Keto, I was constantly tired, never having any energy and my mind was foggy. Once I started doing Keto, I had this new energy that I could tap into and it felt and still feels amazing! My mind is much clearer and I no longer feel tired and I am in a better mood most days. Another benefit is you will tend to stay fuller a lot longer, and you will not feel the need to snack as often.

SO, WHAT IS THIS THIS KETO **DIET?**

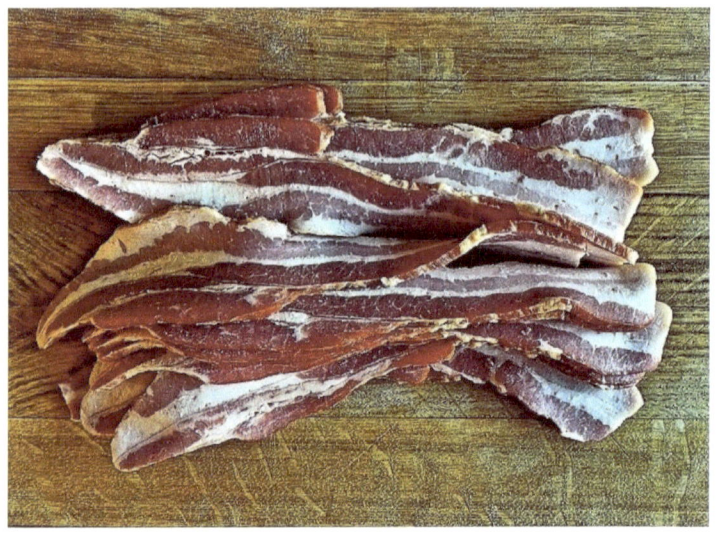

How to Get Into Ketosis, the Lazy Way

Here are the Simple steps on how to get into Ketosis
1. Cut the Carbs PeriodT!!!

If you want to get into Ketosis and stay in Ketosis you will have to cut your carb intake down to **50-100 grams per day**. Say goodbye to Bread, Rice, ect but trust me it will be totally worth if once you start seeing the results!

Below is an example to show you the Lazy way for counting your Carbs for the day. You take the Total Carbohydrate 4 Grams – Dietary Fiber 3 Grams = 1 Net Carb. If there is not any dietary Fiber, just count the Total Carbohydrate. As long as you are between 50-100 grams in a day, you are Golden!!

NUTRITION FACTS

3 servings per container

Serving size
Amount per serving
Cholesterol 0mg

Sodium 0mg

Total Carbohydrate 4g

   Dietary Fiber 3g

4 Grams- 3 Grams= 1 Net Carb + 3 Servings=
3 Total Net Carbs

2. To get into Ketosis Faster, take some Keto supplements. There is an abundance of Keto supplements from your local Grocery store or on Amazon. These supplements help your body get into Keto a lot faster. We are talking about as fast as in an hour of consumption!

One of the supplements that I recommend, is Insta Ketones by Julian Bakery. It is a powder drink that you can consume with or without caffeine and it does wonders! It may not taste all great, but it gets the job done. I have lost up to 5 to 7 pounds in one week, just drinking it every morning at work with my coffee, this product by far, gets the job done!

Simple Signs That You Are In Ketosis Yay!!

1. You start seeing your numbers drop on the scale. You are looking good over there!!
2. Loss of Appetite and less cravings
3. Increased Focus and Energy
4. Short term Fatigue (We will get into the Keto Flu, don't worry)
5. Dry mouth and increased thirst
6. Increased Ketones – There are plenty of Ketone strips that you can purchase at your local store such as Walgreens or Amazon that you can use to test how much Ketones you have in your body, at any point of time.

LAZY KETO. THE SIMPLE GUIDE TO LOSE WEIGHT THE LAZY WAY.

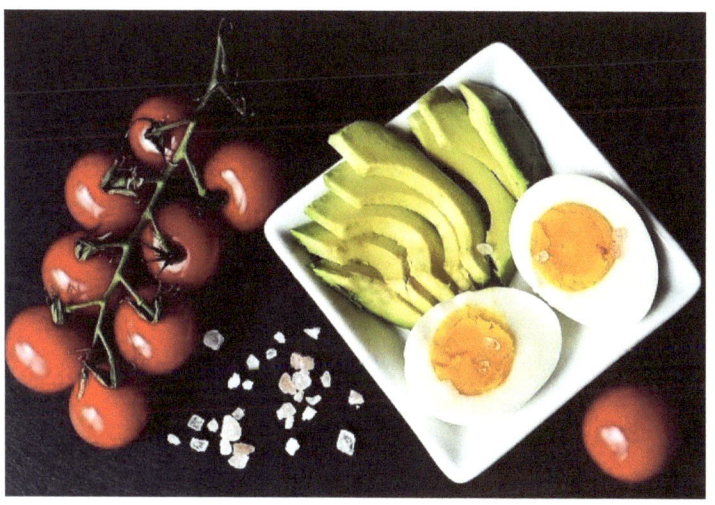

What is the Keto Flu?

The Keto Flu Too Shall Pass

The **Keto Flu** is not the big bad wolf and is not as bad as it sounds. Switching from a high-carb diet to a low-carb diet life style lowers insulin levels in your body. This is healthy and one of the ultimate goals of a Ketogenic diet. When insulin levels are low, your liver begins converting your fat into ketones, which most of your cells can use in place of glucose.

Keto Flu is your body's reaction, when adjusting to the Keto Diet. Your body is being forced to use Ketones as energy, rather than your normal glucose. These symptoms tend to happen your first week on Keto. They can last up to two weeks, but everyone's body is different. Here are the most common Keto Flu symptoms:

- Fatigue
- Headache
- Irritability
- Muscle cramps
- Dizziness

- Lack of motivation
- Dry mouth, Dehydration

Do not be alarmed as the keto flu too shall pass! My experience, the first few days weas having a headache, irritability, and feeling fatigue. But again, everyone is different. This is just a temporary thing and you will be feeling awesome and looking like a million dollars in no time!

The Cure for the Keto Flu

Here are a few things that will help your body adapt and get over these temporary symptoms in no time.

1. **Stay hydrated.** Drinking a lot of water in your first week about 6 to 8 cups a day can help reduce your body from fatigue and with irritability.

2. **Take vitamins.** Replace your electrolytes taking supplements such as Magnesium Citrate and multi vitamins, that you can purchase at your local grocery store. Also try to increase your sodium levels by adding Sea salt to your Keto meals or you can drink bone broth soup. To keep your potassium and magnesium in check, try eating nuts, seeds (in moderation), fish, and dark leafy greens.

3. **Get Plenty of Sleep.** Make sure you are getting 7 to 8 hours of sleep. With lack of sleep, your keto flu symptoms, may become worse due to cortisol levels increasing because of the lack of sleep. So get that beauty sleep!

4. **Do not restrict your calorie intake the first week.** Eat until you feel full. Your appetite will start to decrease, once your body starts adapting to the your new Keto life style. So relax, enjoy that bacon and eggs and try not to over think it.

5. **Lay off the physical activity.** I know, I know this is

probably obvious as this is the lazy guide. Just thought I would throw this in for fun☺.

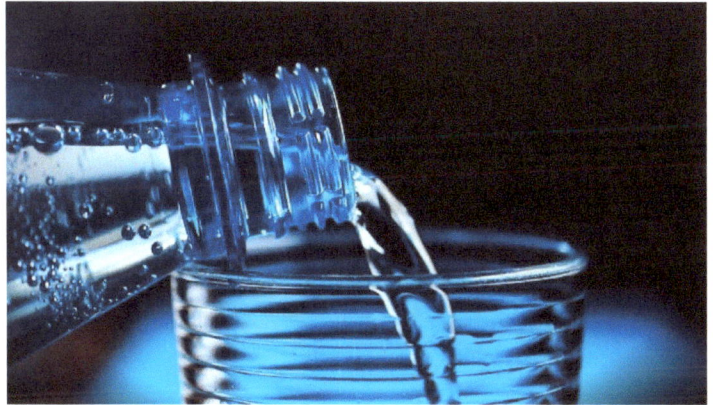

Please don't tell me, I have to work out to lose weight.

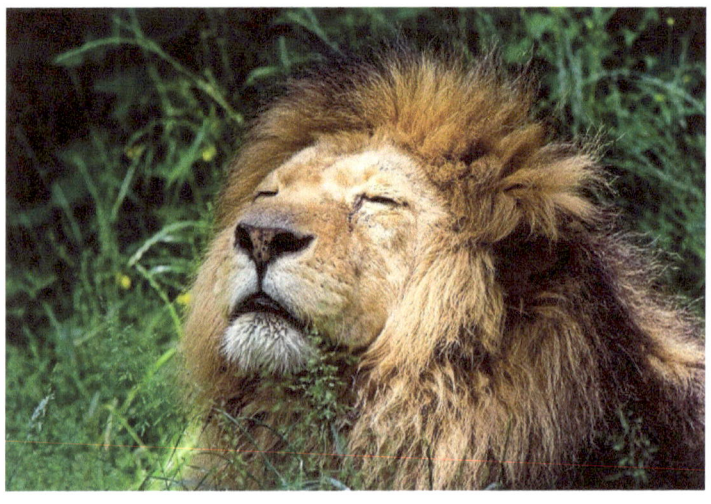

The main question that I get asked all the time when people notice my weight loss and I talk to them about my Keto weight loss success, is always did you have to work out? Or do you work out? It's simply, no. You will lose weight on keto simply by sticking to your new eating habits and your new keto life style. It's as easy as that, period. If you want to work out, by all means knock yourself out. However, in my three years of trials and tribulations on keto, working out and not working out, I personally did not see that much of a difference with working out. I worked out for a few months when I first started Keto in 2016 and I averaged about one pound per week, which is the same amount of weight, I was losing without working out.

[1]Again, this is based on my own personal experience. If you stick to this plan, you will lose weight without needing to work out.

---

[1] Image by <a href="https://pixabay.com/users/27707-27707/?utm_source=link-attribution&utm_medium=referral&utm_campaign=image&utm_con ten Phillips</a> from <a href="https://pixabay.com/?utm_source=link-attribution&utm_medium=referral&utm_campaign=im-age&utm_content=951778">Pixabay</a>

2.Image by <a href="https://pixabay.com/users/congerdesign-509903/?utm_source=link-attribution&utm_medium=refer-ral&utm_campaign=image&utm_content=2032980">co n- gerdesign</a> from <a href="https://pixabay.com/?utm_source=link-attribution&utm_medium=referral&utm_campaign=im-age&utm_content=2032980">Pixabay</a>

3. Image by <a href="https://pixabay.com/users/Wokandapix-614097/?utm_source=link-attribution&utm_medium=refer-ral&utm_campaign=image&utm_content=2372177">W okan- dapix</a> from <a href="https://pixabay.com/?utm_source=link-attribution&utm_medium=referral&utm_campaign=im-age&utm_content=2372177">Pixabay</a>
4. Image by <a href="https://pixabay.com/users/zuzyusa-6383069/?utm_source=link-attribution&utm_medium=re-

ferral&utm_campaign=image&utm_con-
tent=3223286">zuzyusa</a>   from   <a
        href="https://pix- abay.com/?utm_source=link-
attribution&utm_medium=refer-
ral&utm_campaign=image&utm_content=3223286">Pix
- abay</a>

I have managed to lose over 70 pounds in the course of three years, just by sticking to my keto eating habits (for the most part, will go into detail later) and not having to go to the gym every single day. If you stick to the diet, by tracking your net carbs every day, you can also get these type of results.

The Overall Goal

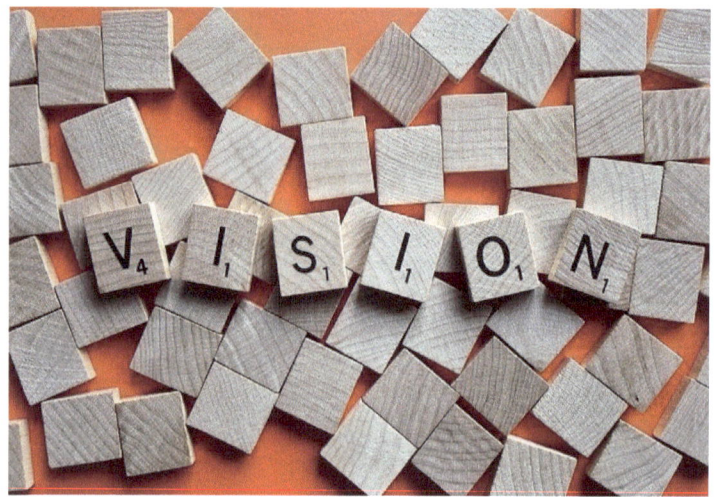

So, the overall goal to maintaining your lazy but awesome Keto lifestyle is the easiest yet hardest part, sticking to it!!! If you cheat, and I am speaking from experience from my trials and errors here, you will automatically kick your body out of ketosis. Once you kick your body out of ketosis, which is using your fat to burn fat, you will have to start <u>ALL OVER AGAIN</u>. Yes, that means going thru that crappy Keto Flu again… Trust me, you do not want to do this. I made this bad decision on a trip to Disneyland with my boyfriend.

After adopting my lazy keto lifestyle, seeing results on a weekly basis, getting closer to my ultimate goal weight, which was in arms reach, and I decided, "hey why not cheat a little, I am at the happiest place on earth right?". Wrong Idea!!! Not only did I gain 10 pounds on this carb eating frenzy, it was harder for me to get back on track into my lazy keto routine. Not only that, but I literally felt like crap, mentally and physically. I had no energy, was very moody, and it sucked very very much! Bottom line if you decide to cheat and just have that one cookie, donut, churro, or whatever, it's a lot harder to get back on and stay the course.

After your body is in Ketosis, you want to count your carbs but also watch your calorie intake. There are many websites and apps that will provide you with your daily calorie goals to assist you on your weight loss Journey. I recommend tracking your food intake on apps like Lose it and My fitness Pal the first few months. After that, you will have a good idea what's good and not good for you to eat.

Please learn from my setbacks, so that you do not have to do the same thing as me. The key here, is to commit to this as a
Lazy Keto Lifestyle. I say lifestyle, because you have to look at it as not as some fad diet, a trend, or something you do to lose a couple of pounds and go back to your old eating habits. Because if you do, you will gain back all or most of the weight you lost and this will all be for nothing and we do not want that do we? I

want you to have the best results and have an awesome success story. If you are willing to make this a lifestyle choice and stick to your new plan, you will see results. So, now ask yourself, are you ready for this Journey?

Food List

Below is a list of foods that are Keto friendly:

- Bacon and Sausage
- Beef
- Pork
- Poultry
- Fish and seafood
- Eggs
- Natural fat, high-fat sauces
- High-fat dairy such as Butter, Cheese, Sour Cream, High fat Yogurts in moderation
- Unsweetened almond milk, try to avoid Milk.
- Nuts such as Pecans, Brazil nuts and macadamia nuts
- Berries such Blueberries, strawberries, ect (In Moderation)
- Whip Cream
- Dark chocolate 7o% to 90% Ghirardelli is my go to
- Coffee
- Tea without sugar
- Avocados
- Olive Oil
- Coconut Oil
- MCT Oil

- Cocoa Butter

Weight Loss Journey Photos Before

In these photos, I was at my largest between 240 pounds to 230 pounds. I was miserable, tired, out of breathe, fed up, and hiding behind my smiles.

Before & Starting my Keto Journey

LAZY KETO. THE SIMPLE GUIDE TO LOSE WEIGHT THE LAZY WAY.

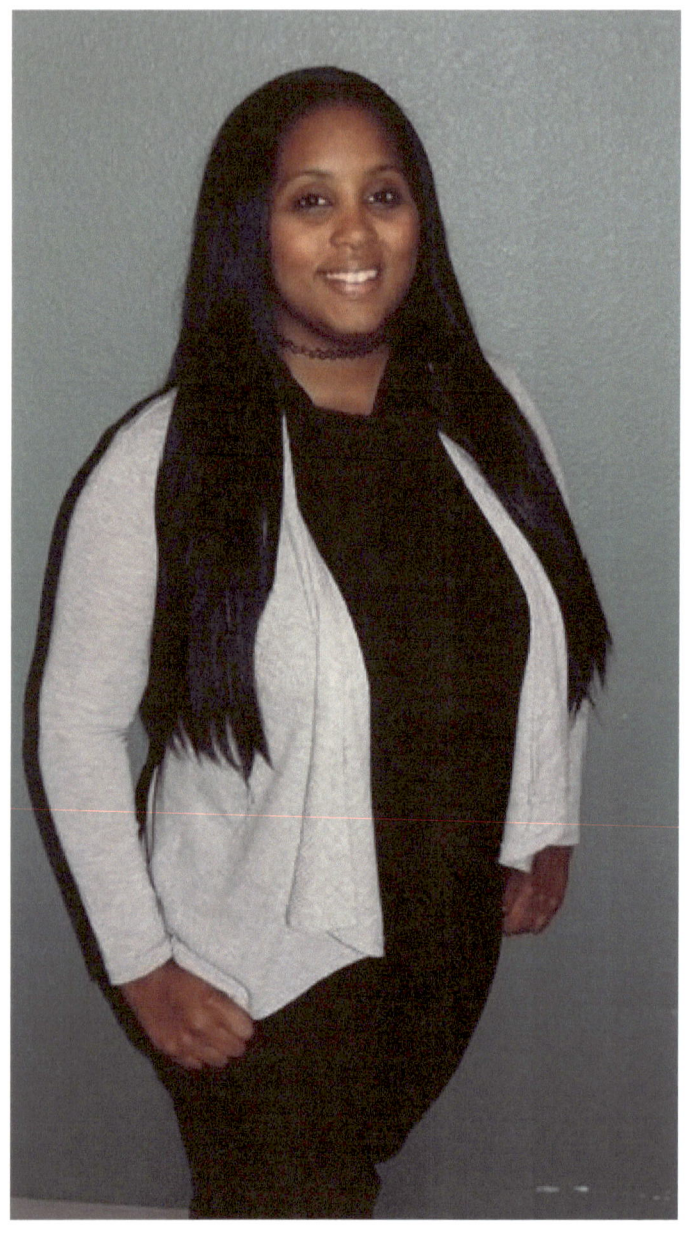

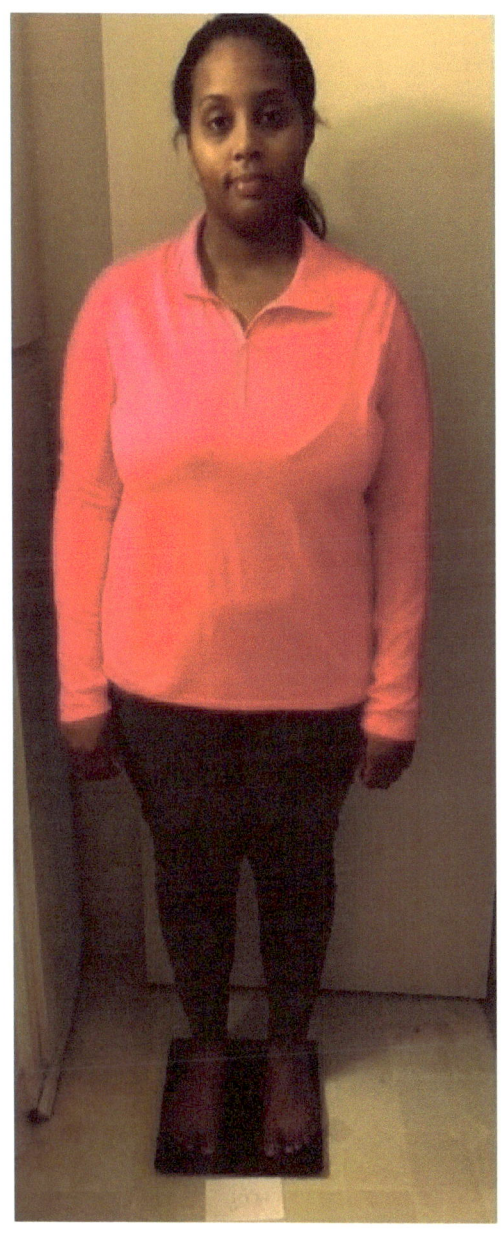

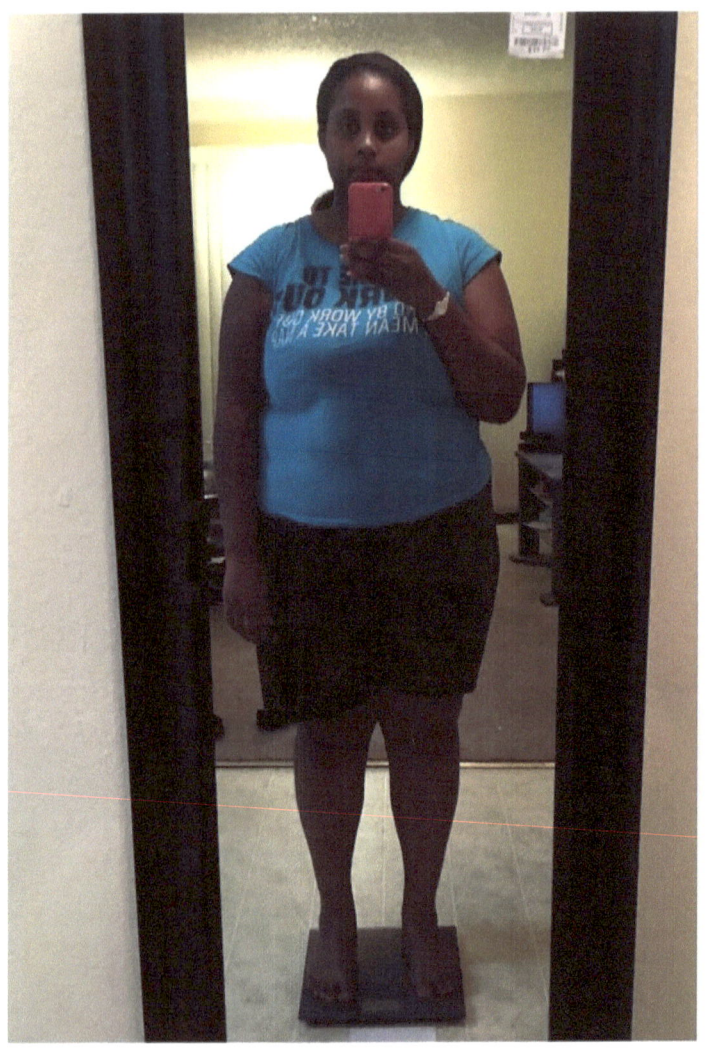

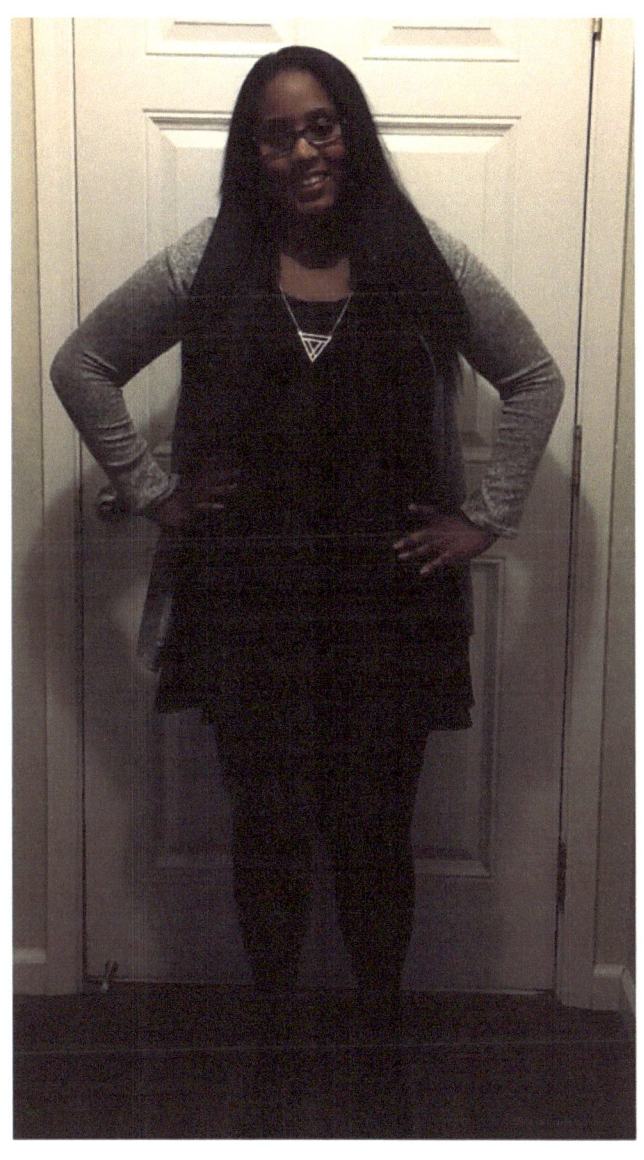

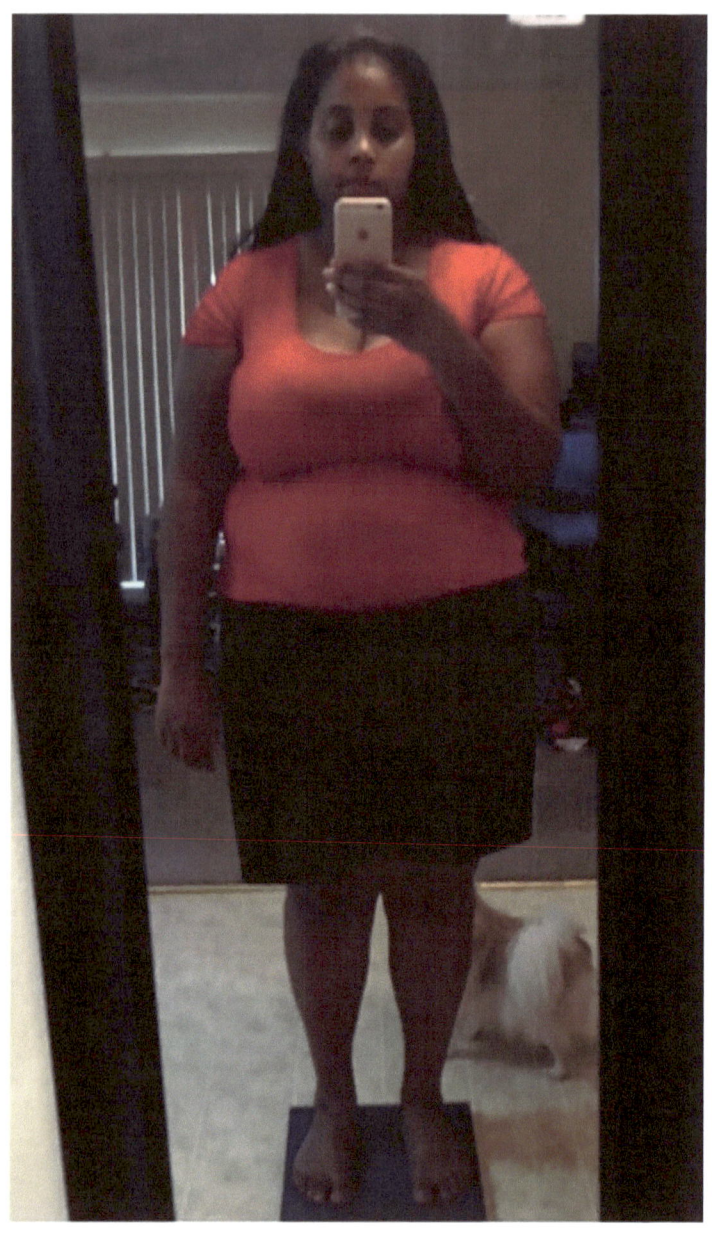

Weight Loss Journey Photos After & Current

Currently down over 70 pounds from a size 16/18 to a size 6/8!! I am still on my weight loss journey with 10 to 15 more pounds to lose, in order to reach my ultimate goal weight.

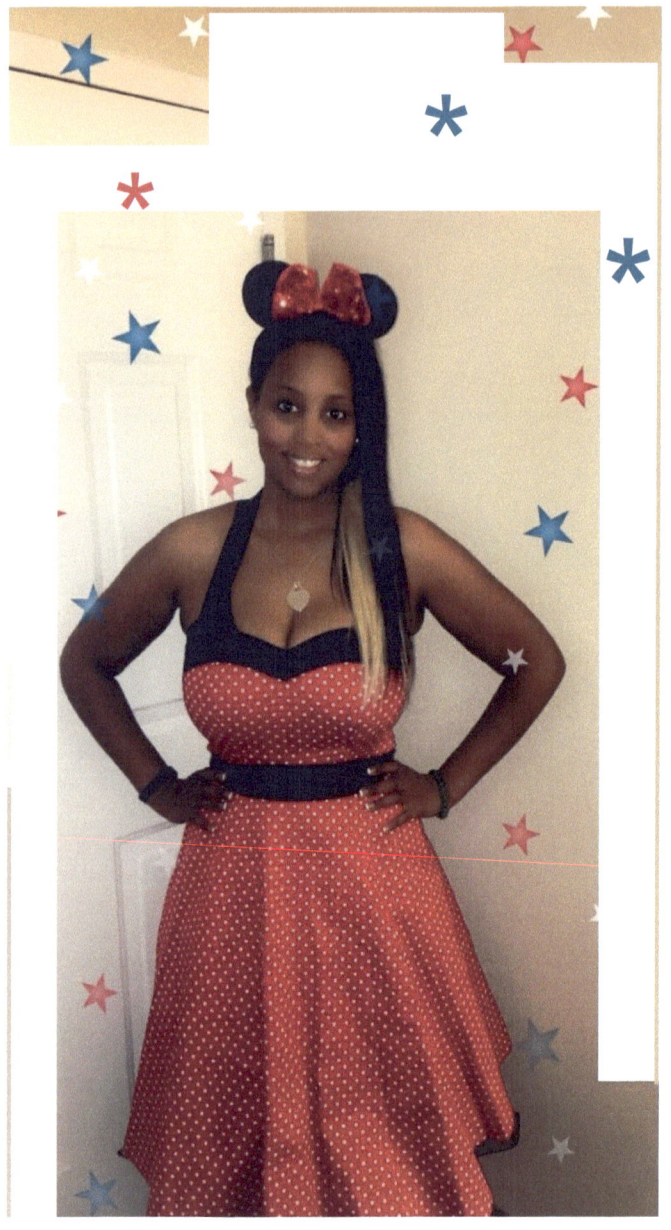

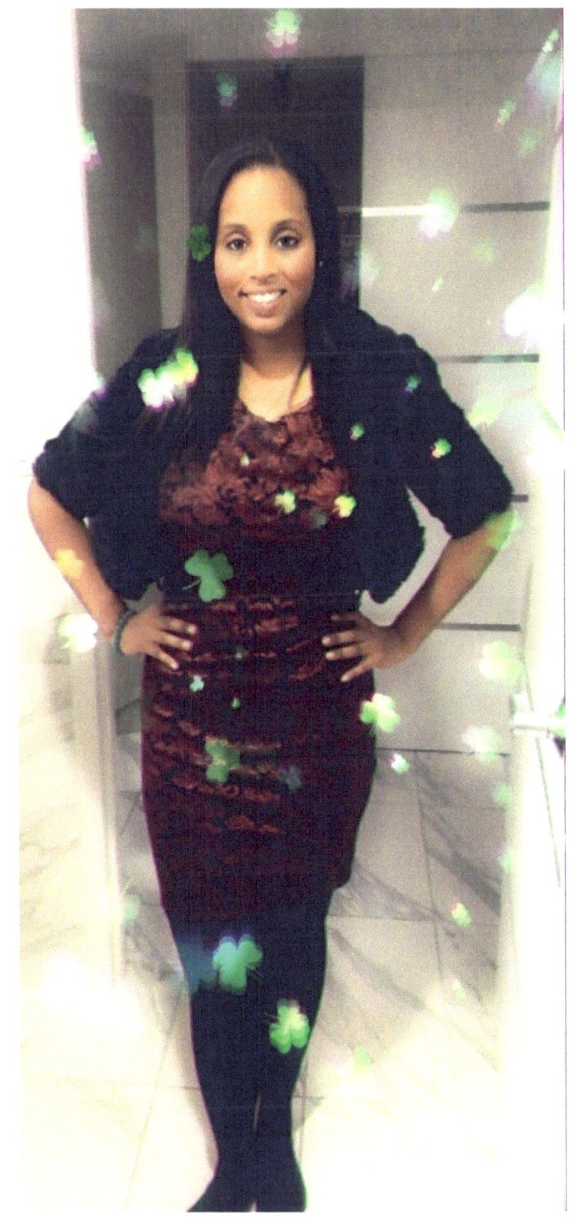

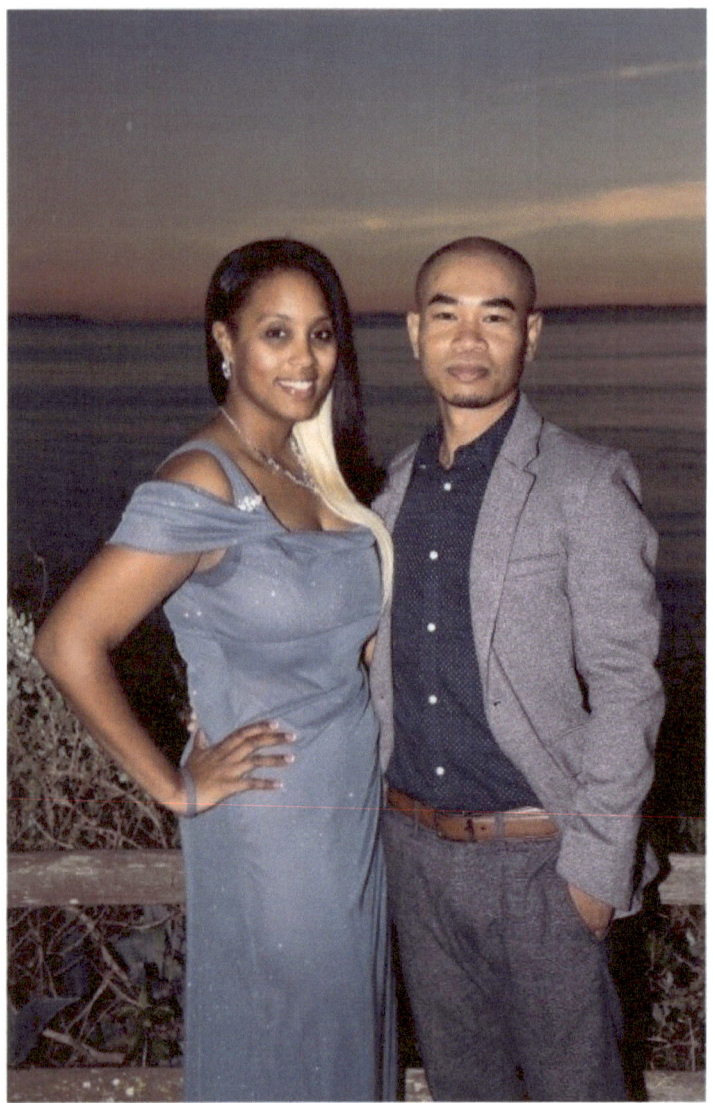

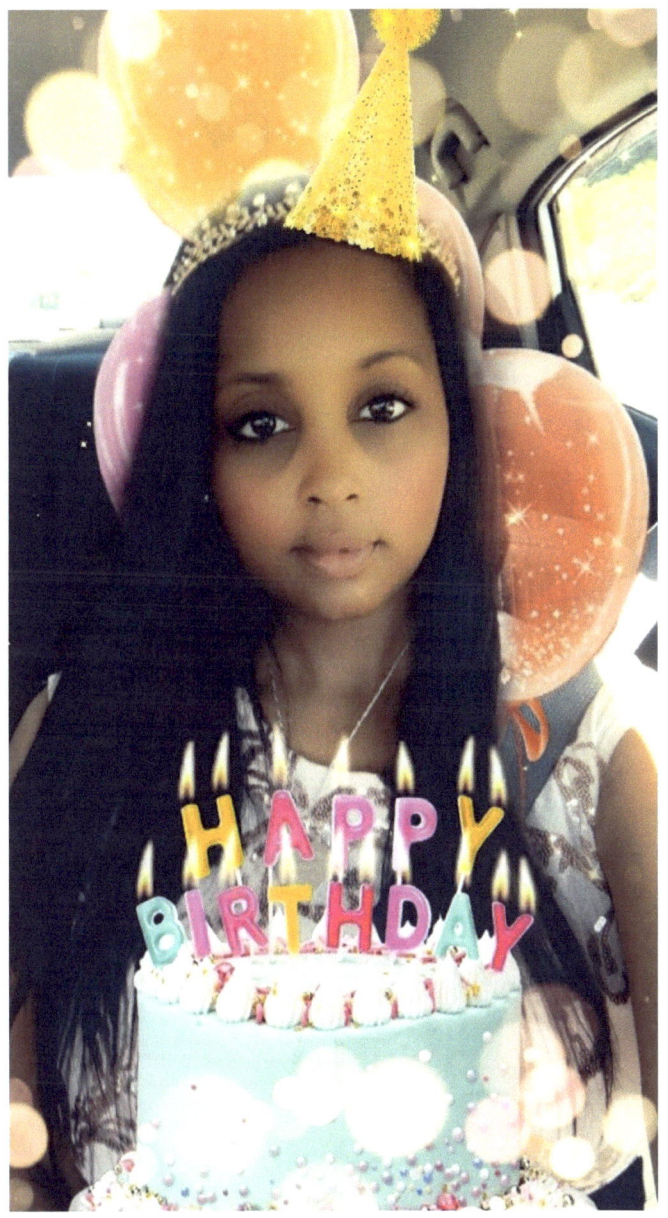

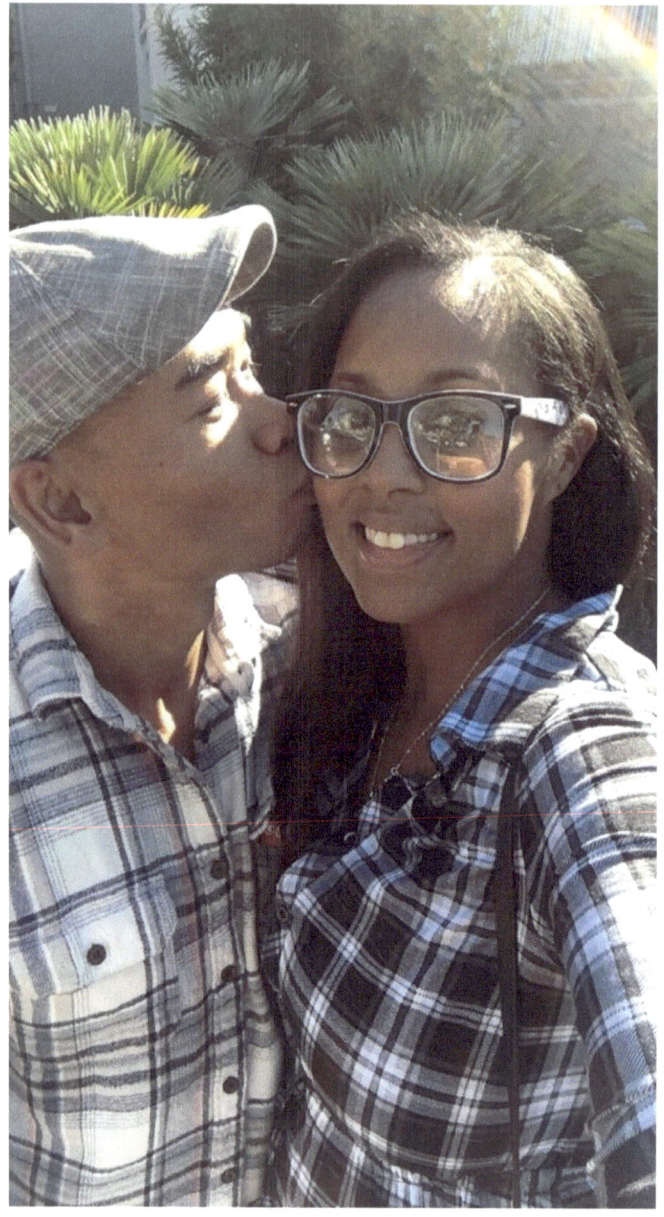

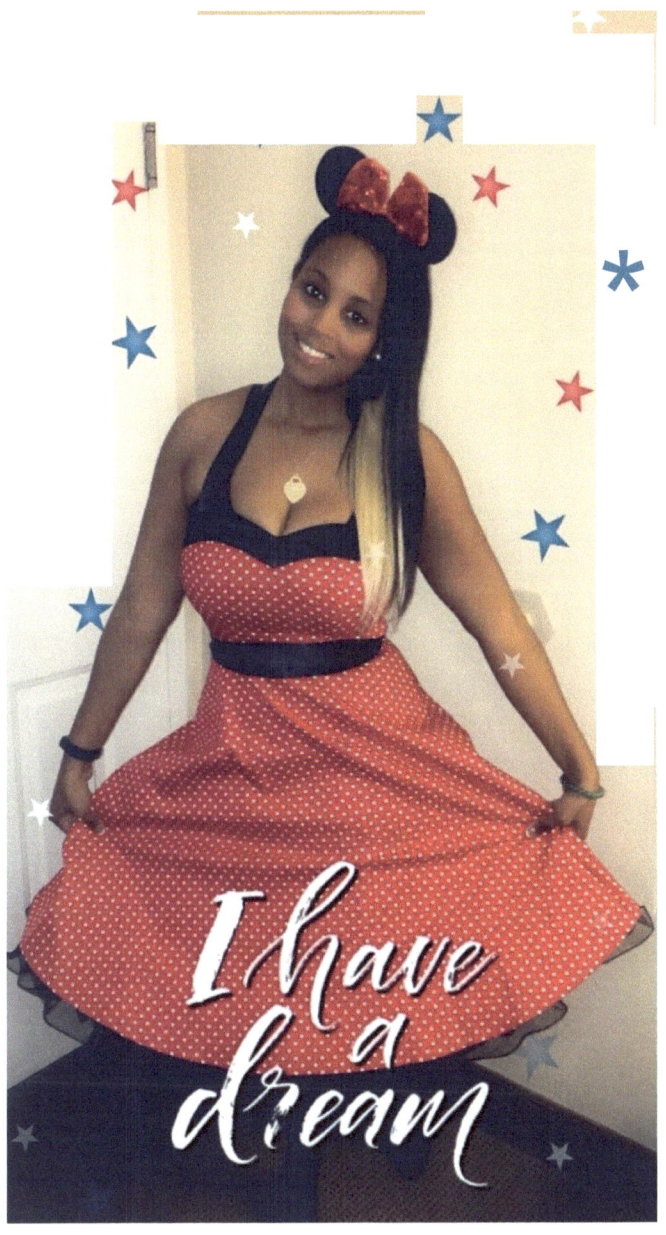

Epilogue

This is only the beginning. Stay tuned and I will continue to guide you with more tips and steps on how to achieve the lazy keto lifestyle and continue to see results, in my next book coming soon. In the meantime feel free to check out my website https://eccentricbeauty422.wixsite.com/ashleysbliss

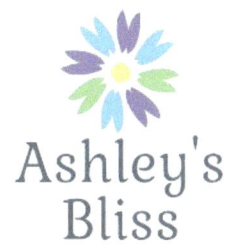

Ashley's
Bliss

About the Author

Ashley Perkins is the founder of Ashley's Bliss Health and Beauty.
What started as a last chance for hope, has now grown into a Keto
Lifestyle. With over 70 pounds lost, she lives and breathes Keto,
Wellness, and overall a Healthy life Balance. She currently resides
in Northern California, with her baby Pomeranian, Paris and
Boyfriend Ray. Visit her at
https://eccentricbeauty422.wixsite.com/ashleysbliss

You can connect with me on:

https://eccentricbeauty422.wixsite.com/ashleysbliss